Ultimate Keto S

Beginners guide to shopping food and drink to their ketogenic diet

By: Dane Louise

Table of Content

MEAT	6
SEAFOOD	8
DAIRY	10
VEGETABLES	12
FRUIT	13
NUTS AND SEEDS	14
OILS AND FATS	15
BAKED GOODS	16
SWEETENERS	17
CONDIMENTS	18
BEVERAGES	20
KETO-FRIENDLY SNACKS	21
WHAT DO WE AVOID?	22

Keto Shopping List

Keto's huge right now. The keto, or ketogenic, diet is quickly becoming one of the hottest diets this year, with tons of claimed benefits from weight loss to fighting cancer, but what is it? And what can and can't you eat on a keto diet?

The keto diet is a low-carb, high-fat diet that offers many health benefits. The whole idea is to reduce carbohydrate intake, replacing carbs with fat. Once you do this, your body goes into a metabolic state called ketosis, which is super efficient at burning fat for energy.

A standard ketogenic diet (SKD) typically contains 75% fat, 20% protein, and 5% carbs. There are tons of studies showing it can help you lose weight and improve overall health, as well as promising research into keto's benefits against diabetes, cancer, epilepsy, and Alzheimer's disease.

So, now you know the science behind it. But what type of foods fit into the keto diet, and what should you put on your keto shopping list? Here's a handy keto-friendly grocery list you can take to the store.

I've grouped the list into the main food groups:

- **Meat**
- **Seafood**
- **Dairy**
- **Vegetables**
- **Fruit**
- **Nuts and seeds**
- **Oils and fats**
- **Baked goods**
- **Sweeteners**

- **Condiments**
- **Beverages**
- **Keto snacks**

Meat

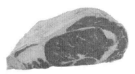

Meat is high in protein and fat and low in carbs, so perfect for a keto diet. If you can, try to get grass-fed, free-range meat when you can.

- **Red meat:**
  - BACON
  - BEEF
  - GAME
  - HAM
  - HOTDOGS
  - LAMB
  - ORGAN MEATS
  - PORK
  - SAUSAGE
  - STEAK
  - VEAL

- **Poultry:**
  - goose
  - chicken
  - duck
  - turkey

- whole birds, drumsticks, breasts, or ground meat for burgers, meatballs, chillis, etc

- **Eggs:**
  - free-range, pastured, or omega-3 whole eggs, Egg Yolks.

Seafood

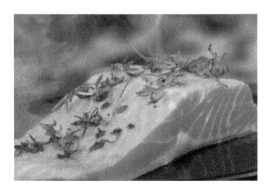

Fish is full of protein, healthy fats, and essential oils like omega-3, making it a perfect addition to your keto shopping list

- **Fatty fish:(Fattier fish is better)**
    - Anchovies
    - Atfish
    - Cod
    - Halibut
    - Herring
    - Mackerel
    - Mackerel
    - Mahi-mahi
    - Salmon
    - Trout
    - Tuna

- **Shellfish:**
  - clams
  - muscles
  - oysters
- **Crustaceans:**
  - Crab
  - crayfish
  - lobsters
  - mussels
  - octopus
  - oysters
  - prawns
  - scallops
  - shrimps
  - squid

Dairy

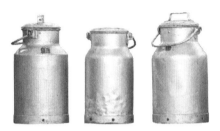

While you won't be able to drink cow's milk on a keto diet, due to its high sugar content, but dairy is not off the table. Butter, cream, and plenty of cheeses have high-fat content and few carbs, so they're perfect for a keto shopping list.

- **Butter/cream**
  - grass-fed if possible

- **Cheese**
  - blue
  - Brie
  - buffalo mozzarella
  - camembert
  - cheddar
  - colby
  - cream
  - mascarpone goat's cheese
  - muenster
  - parmesan
  - provolone

- Swiss
- **Milk**
  - almond
  - cashew
  - coconut
  - flax
  - half-and-half
  - heavy cream
  - pea
  - soy

Vegetables

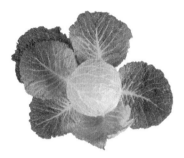

Make sure you get plenty of veggies no matter what diet you're on, but especially on the keto diet. Keep an eye out for low-carb, non-starchy vegetables like greens but avoid root veggies like sweet potatoes and beets, as well as corn.

- **Greens**
  - cabbage
  - collard greens
  - kale
  - lettuce
  - microgreens
  - spinach
- **Broccoli**
- **Cauliflower**
- **Onions**
- **Peppers**
- **Zucchini**

Fruit

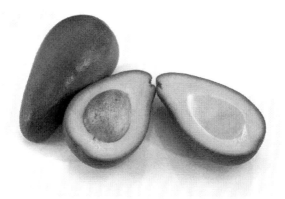

Because most fruits have high sugar content, you'll want to reduce your fruit intake on a keto diet. However, there are a couple of fruits that are perfect for your ketogenic shopping list.

- **Avocado**
- **Cantaloup**
- **Lemons**
- **Peaches**
- **Strawberries**
- **Tomatoes**
- **Watermelon**

Nuts and seeds

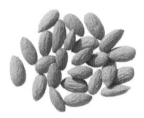

Nuts and seeds will quickly become your best friends on a ketogenic diet. They're perfect for getting protein and healthy oils and fats into your main courses, salads, and snacks. Due to their high-fat and low-carb content, you'll want plenty of nuts and seeds on your keto grocery list.

- **Almonds**
- **Brazil nuts**
- **Chia seeds**
- **Flax seeds**
- **Hazelnuts**
- **Hemp seeds**
- **Macadamia nuts**
- **Pecans**
- **Pumpkin seeds**
- **Sunflower seeds**
- **Walnuts**

Oils and fats

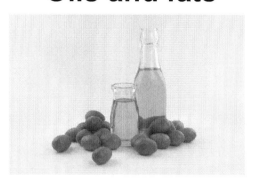

Every diet needs a good source of oils and fats. The keto diet promotes high fat intake, so make sure you're getting your oils and fats from healthy sources. Unhealthy fats can wreak havoc on your body, so this is a key section to your shopping list for a keto diet. Try to avoid unhealthy fats like vegetable oil and mayonnaise.

- Avocado oil
- Butter and ghee (non-hydrogenated)
- Cocoa Butter
- Coconut Butter
- Coconut oil
- Duck fat
- Extra virgin olive oil
- Hazelnut oil
- lard
- nut oils
- schmaltz
- Sesame oil
- tallow

Baked goods

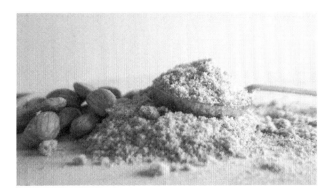

A keto diet doesn't mean you're going to have to stop eating bread and other tasty baked goods. All you have to do is replace the wheat flour with low-carb alternatives.

- **Almond flour**
- **Coconut flour**
- **Psyllium husk powder**

Sweeteners

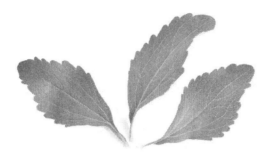

Most sweeteners are high in sugar content, i.e., carbs, so beware of the common sweeteners like honey, palm sugar, maple syrup, Splenda, agave syrup, and coconut sugar. Instead, look for the following sweeteners to add to your grocery list for keto.

- **Cocoa powder**
- **Stevia:**
  - natural, plant-based sweetener with no calories or carbs
- **Sucralose**
  - artificial sweetener
- **Sugar alcohols**
  - naturally-occurring sweeteners like erythritol and xylitol
- **Monk fruit sweetener**
  - plant-based sweetener from China

Condiments

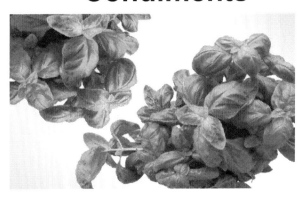

You're going to have to say goodbye to ketchup, mustard, BBQ sauce, and most of your favorite processed condiments when you start your keto diet. Instead, you can make your own using herbs, spices, salt, pepper, and a little olive oil.

- **Salt and pepper**
- **Herbs**
  - basil
  - cilantro
  - dill
  - mint
  - parsley
  - rosemary
  - sage
  - thyme
- **Spices**
  - chili powder
  - cinnamon
  - cloves

- cumin

- curry powder

- garlic powder

- paprika

Beverages

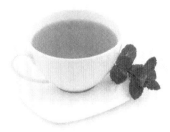

Plenty of common drinks out there are high in sugar and carbs. Beer, spirits, soda, energy drinks, milkshakes, and juice are all no-gos on keto. Instead, look for unsweetened, diet alternatives.

- **Water:** still and sparkling

- **Black tea**

- **Coconut water**

- **Coffee**

- **Diet soda**

- **Green tea**

- **Unsweetened dairy alternatives:** almond milk, coconut milk, etc.

Keto-friendly snacks

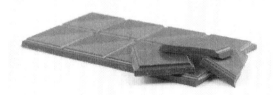

We all love to snack throughout the day, and it looks like snacking between meals is a great way to lose weight. Many common snacks, like potato chips, chocolate, and candy, aren't suitable for keto diets because of their high carb contents. Instead, here are some of my favorite keto-friendly alternatives to graze on throughout the day.

- **Nuts and seeds**

- **Cheese and olives**

- **Hardboiled eggs**

- **Dark chocolate:** at least 70% cocoa content

- **Low-carb shakes:** unsweetened almond milk, cocoa powder, and peanut butter

- **Celery with guacamole**

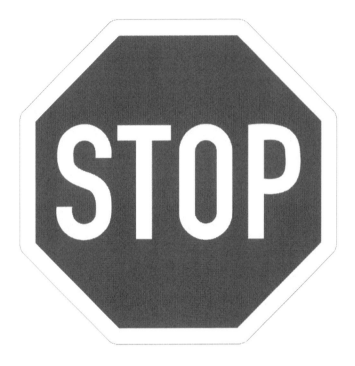

What do we avoid?

There are also a few foods you'll need to avoid on a keto diet:

- **Sugary food**

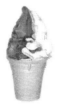

  - Candy
  - fruit juice
  - ice cream
  - soda‹etc

- **Sweeteners**

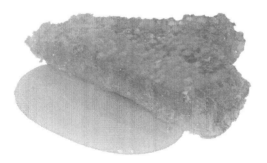

  - agave nectar
  - dates
  - Honey

- Maltodextrin
- maple syrup

- **Grains and starches**

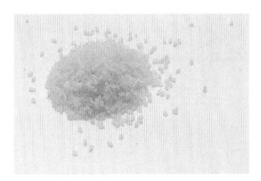

- bread
- cereal
- pasta
- Rice, etc

- **Fruit: Fruit is very high in sugar**

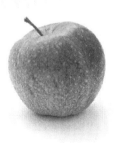

- **Beans and legumes**

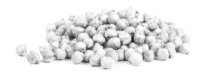

  - Lentils
  - butter beans
  - chickpeas
  - kidney beans
  - peas, etc.

- **Root vegetables and tubers**

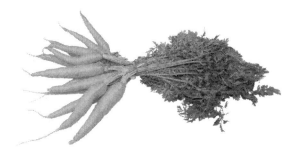

  - Carrots
  - parsnips

- potatoes
- sweet potatoes, etc

- **Cow's milk:**
  - Milk contains lactose, a type of sugar, and is high in carbs

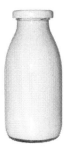

- **Alcohol:**
  - Most alcoholic beverages have high carb contents

- **Processed food:**
  - Most processed food is high in sugar

Printed in Great Britain
by Amazon

15970443R00016